"Stephen Drew
It is wonder full.
one would want
took me into exi‿   ‿‿‿‿‿‿. ɪ ̃o ̃better thing can a
writer do! Bravo."

—GUNILLA NORRIS, AUTHOR OF *CALLING THE CREATURES*

"This book is a gift to anyone who has encountered, or will encounter, death–that is to say, everyone alive. I was left with my own wondering very much intact, and I'm grateful for the author's insights into this mystery that connects us all. "

—HEIDI BARR, AUTHOR OF *COLLISIONS OF EARTH AND SKY*

"With a tender honesty, in prose reminiscent of an old friend's voice, Stephen Drew offers up '...the role of death as a portal to something wondrous,' inviting us to wonder about death along with him in this short and marvelous book that is as much a *memento mori* as it is memoir. If we are to follow Hemingway's instruction to 'write what you know,' Drew has done just that. *Around the Forever Bend* is a great reminder that we can choose to see death as 'an oddly familiar, omniscient teacher,' It reminds us, too, how our contemplation of death can vitalize our relationship to life, how grief changes yet never leaves us completely, and how we might approach our own death with an open heart, until '...our dream here is set aside as we awaken to what follows.'"

—C.M. RIVERS, AUTHOR OF *HOW TO CARRY SOUP*

AROUND THE FOREVER BEND

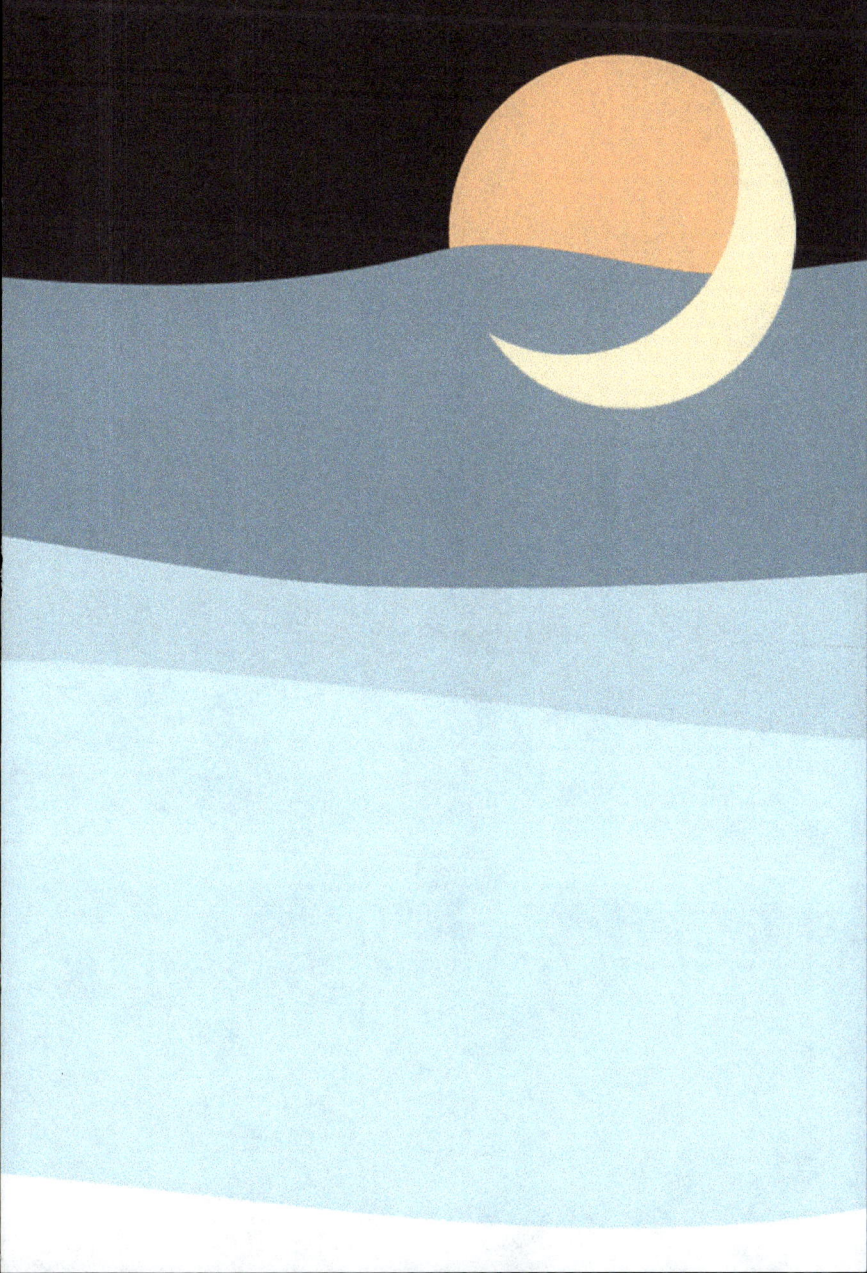

AROUND THE FOREVER BEND

*Remembrances of Wondering
What Lies Beyond Death*

STEPHEN DREW

HOMEBOUND PUBLICATIONS
BERKSHIRE MOUNTAINS, MASS.

LITTLE BOUND BOOKS
WWW.HOMEBOUNDPUBLICATIONS.COM

© 2023 TEXT BY STEPHEN DREW

Little Bound Books support copyright. Copyright fuels creativity, encourages diverse voices, promotes free speech, and creates a vibrant culture. Thank you for buying an authorized edition of this book and for complying with copyright laws by not reproducing, scanning, or distributing any part of it in any form without permission. You are supporting writers and allowing us to continue to publish books for every reader.

All Rights Reserved

Published in 2022 by Little Bound Books

Cover Design and Interior Design by Leslie M. Browning

Interior Art: Dasha "Museberry" from Odessa, Ukraine

ISBN 978-1-956368-20-8

First Edition Trade Paperback

10 9 8 7 6 5 4 3 2 1

Homebound Publications and its imprint, Little Bound Book, is committed to ecological stewardship. We greatly value the natural environment and invest in conservation. For each book purchased in our online store we plant one tree.

PO Box 1601, Northampton, MA 01060	
860.574.5847	info@homeboundpublications.com

HOMEBOUNDPUBLICATIONS.COM & WAYFARERBOOKS.ORG

ALSO BY THE AUTHOR

Into the Thin:
A Pilgrimage Walk Across Northern Spain

for the folks
for the boys
for all who've wondered

———————

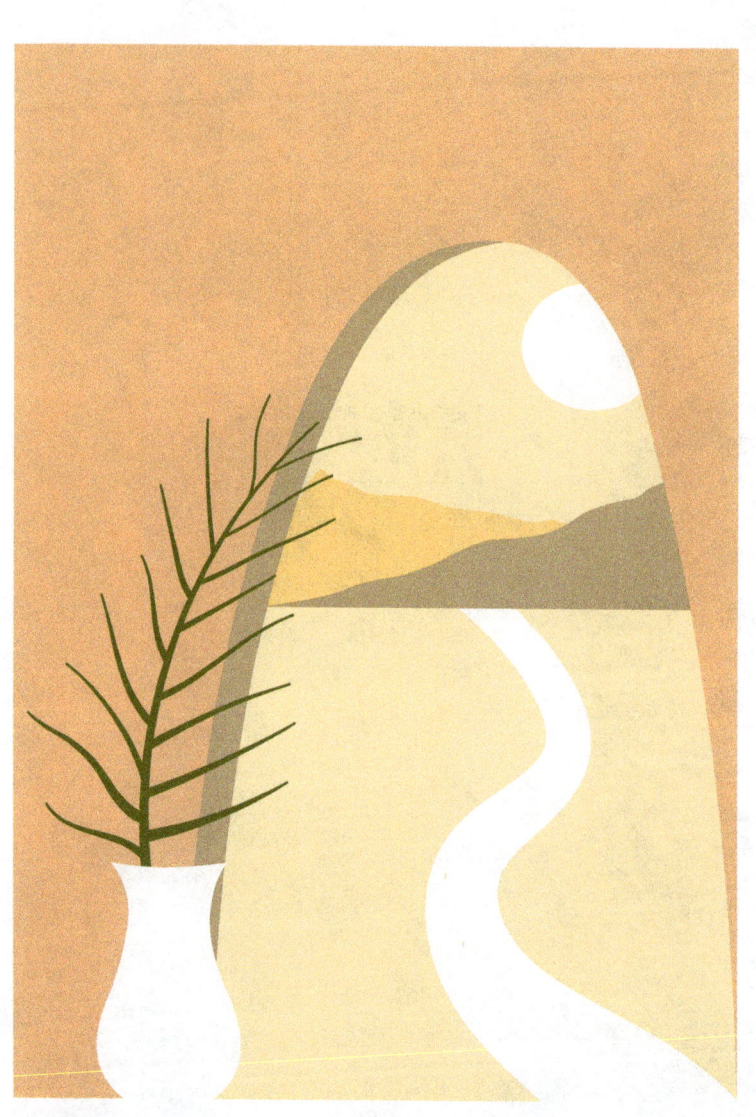

AUTHOR'S NOTE

It was during a lull in the production schedule of my first book when the opening scene of this one came to mind. I was alone on a long drive heading to southern Virginia, and just east of Chesapeake Bay, it jumped up off the road. I knew there was something to it. I also knew it was going to be a short work, a lyrical essay of sorts, and I wanted to be brief—mostly to see if I could. It's a surprisingly hard thing to do, more so when the words are centered on matters of death, matters that have unfolded over a lifetime. One must necessarily leave some things between the lines.

It is mostly in the interest of this desire for brevity that what follows is not comprehensive. I've kept some things to myself, and others I've written of elsewhere. It's not about volume. It's about putting thoughts forth to the page, something to be passed along. In this case, a note of gratitude to what has been a great teacher.

While it's true there are many others with more experience as intimate companions to the dead and dying, it seems I've still been able to accrue some understanding of the inherent relationship between life and death, and how one informs the other. I find this comforting regardless of whether I am currently in a state of conscious grieving or not. It is also an understanding that, for me, has nearly eliminated the concept of loss as a synonym for death. More, it has become evidence of a great continuance, all-ness, and only-ness of life.

Here, I offer something to wonder about in the spirit of fearing it just a little less.

A NOTE FOR READERS

Those who have experienced close proximity to death by suicide know well the trauma that can follow and persist. The author counts himself among them. It is with sensitivity to this that the following advisory is offered: Please be aware the book contains a brief but vivid description of such a death.

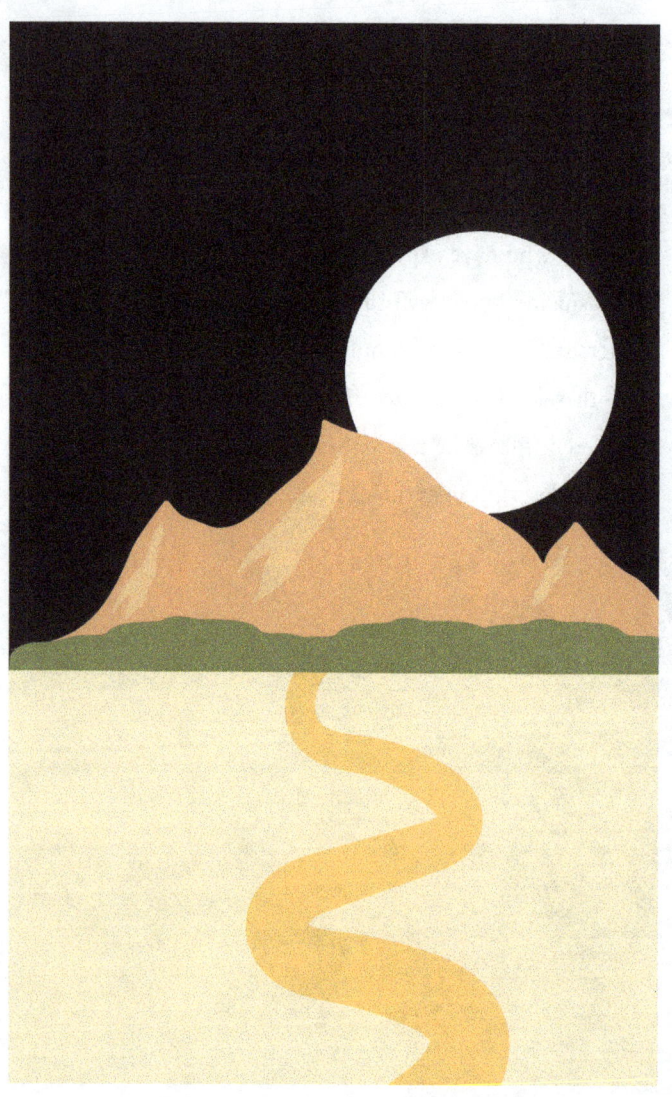

It's around 1:00AM, the ward is dark, and I have the curtains pulled around Jim's bed. I'm seated to his left in an uncomfortable plastic chair which faces the wall behind the bed. My left hand is resting on his left forearm as a connecting point. I have a book in my lap. There is a goose-necked lamp just to my right, its light falling mostly on the book. A generous morphine drip is running, so his breathing is soft and mostly without the gurgle of secretions, his horrific pain abated at least for the moment. There is almost no place on his body which can be touched without touching a tumor.

My shift ended over an hour ago, but I've made a commitment to be here still. As a newly minted Navy Hospital Corpsman, I'm all in. Somehow, it's gotten into my head that no one should die alone. Death is a pretty big deal, the ultimate source of all our fear, the ultimate irreversible moment, the ultimate adventure. So, to have this or any soul take its leave absent of reasonably good company just seems a bit callous to my idealistic 19-year-old mind. Should he pass in the quiet way I'm assuming he will, he'd be found on rounds were he alone. It just wouldn't seem right.

Jim, a retired, 38-year-old Air Force Master Sargent had been admitted to Ward 1-A of the Philadelphia Naval Hospital with end stage cancer. He knew the score. My recollection is he was brought in for palliative care. No available treatment was going to touch this. It was the mid-1970s. Before he reached the last stage of his illness, he would look at me with pleading, agonized eyes, begging to "put me out."

"Come on man," he'd say. "You can do it! Grow some fucking balls and do it!"

"You know I can't, Jim. I can't take your life."

"Then, fuck you."

I'd give him a dose if it was time, the pain would ease, and he'd apologize for being an asshole. I'd tell him he was no asshole—that maybe someday, people would get to choose. I'd also tell him I was honored to be of service to him.

He was heroic when his wife was there, which was every evening. Attempting to modulate his voice and facial expressions, he would valiantly try to hide his pain from her. It was impossible.

His eyes would give him away. Eyes will do that as they become laden and hollow, tortured and crucified. She would leave each night around 9:00 to relieve a friend watching the two little ones at home.

It's impossibly quiet. I'm reading. Jim is breathing. His respirations have been falling off, but regular. The agonal breathing is yet to come, and I sense a long night ahead for us both. He begins to shift a bit, maybe coming up a little from the morphine. I wonder intuitively if something isn't gathering within him, but he settles, and I return to my book. Time passes.

A soft clicking noise lifts from him and interrupts my reading as my attention first goes to my left hand resting on his arm. I note the difference in how it feels. The change has come. My gaze goes from the page to his face, to his eyes, now open slightly and looking just past me. I see an expression of peace and relief, of wonder tinged with awe, and yet utterly absent of animation. Doll's eyes. But could they speak, they would say, "Oh my friend, if you only knew…if only."

*   *   *

It seems to me I've always had an intimate relationship with this page turning we call death. It began when I was a very young child, and as I write now at age 63, it shows no sign of tapering. In fact, this is the stage of life where friends begin to leave. It just happened again a few weeks ago, and it got me to thinking.

I tend to not mourn…at least not in the classic sense of deep sorrow for the departed one, nor am I transported into a period of existential angst which can happen as one ages. More, I wonder. I wonder about what lies beyond the senses. It's been going on for a long time. I suspect it may for some time more.

* * *

On Saturday mornings during my early-to-later childhood, I would be required to play alone in my room while my parents slept in. I was always an early riser on the weekends, free from the dread and loathing of having to endure a day at school. As an only child, it was a time rich in fantasy—my weekly sojourn to the Land of Make Believe (well before Mr. Rogers). It was then I would often interact with my younger siblings; the first, a brother, followed by two sisters, all of whom died at the time of their birth.

I had been somehow made to understand that they had once been alive and real, yet would be no more, ever again. Ever. I'd love to know how I was made to understand this, but I simply have no recollection. It would likely shed some light on how I came to view death. My parents, who were responsible for my understanding, were devoutly Catholic, and I'm sure the imagery of angels on clouds from the illustrated catechism books contributed as well. I learned early on that I could be with them at will even though I had no idea what they looked or sounded like, what sort of personalities they might have developed, what kind of family members they would have become. Left to my imagination, I knew them all intimately. I was their older brother, and I honored my position in our family.

On those Saturday mornings in my room, behind my closed door, with secrecy and silence a mystical experience would take place. Well beyond an exercise in coping with their deaths, I believe it was my very first pathway to a far country, boundless and beautiful and warmly lit like a waking dream. Death itself provided a way in; the very seed of something transcendent. Though of course our relationships have faded with age as my perceptions have changed, today they are no less real to me. They are intrinsic to me still, and so I do not mourn.

I attended wakes during my childhood—family friends, a clergy member, a distant relative. In those days, children were not sheltered from the sight of a dead body in a casket, yet I don't recall having had any nightmares because of this. Mostly, I just wondered. I wondered about the difference between a living person and the obviously non-living person in the box. The deceased always impressed me as appearing like store mannequins, human in shape, but somehow non-human and empty, a husk. Something was missing and I was told it was their soul. Most of the children I knew (Catholic grammar school students all) were content with this explanation, but I was not. I wondered what dead would feel like, laying there dressed in a suit, a rosary strung through my hands, missing something essential. Fortunately, I didn't share this. Parents of only children who have lost others at birth tend to be overprotective. Their trauma induces panic. Still, I remember it as something that occupied its fair share of my thoughts.

And early in the midst of this, President Kennedy was killed.

The nun who was the principal poked her head into our second-grade classroom and motioned toward the nun who was the teacher. There was a brief conference in the hallway, and the sister returned to us, her face as white as her habit. She told us the President had been assassinated, meaning he was now dead. None of us knew what assassinated meant, but we knew in general terms what the word dead suggested. I knew I did. Maybe better than most. The President was now in the same condition as my siblings.

We were sent home, and I walked into my mother's arms just inside the front door. Her upset was palpable, for at the time she was also on the heels of having experienced the second death of a child at birth, a daughter. Now, death was visiting from outside our home. She held me tightly, and then we sat before the TV, watching images and hearing words I could not comprehend. She tried to explain, but it was impossible. All I could intuit was that somehow, very quickly, everything in the world had changed. There had been a catastrophe. I also recalled having the sense that this death was far more important to everyone else than my sister's had been.

Though not as given to emotion as was my mother, my father's mood was subdued as he arrived home later that day. I'm sure he had called her from the office earlier. I have no recollection of their interaction about all of what happened that day, but neither do I recall anything dramatic. Together, they were always quiet about this sort of thing, and most things for that matter. For them, it was more likely a continuation of their own loss, or at least its darkness. As for me, this day and the subsequent outpouring of the nation's collective mourning, informed me of how to regard death and grief—and the power they both would hold.

Within the following year, another and final infant death came upon us, and about it, memory has failed me save for this: My mother blowing kisses to me from the window of her hospital room. It was all we could do. No children were allowed.

When I was 16, a junior in high school, life was a model of sweetness and simplicity. I had a pretty girlfriend, a part time job, and was a track athlete. Though managing reasonably well in my studies, I had decided by this time that I lacked the academic discipline or interest required for college. Military service and job training would, at least for now, be my likely path and I rested in this. The

Saturday morning play dates with my brother and sisters were, of course, long behind me—our contact now primarily experienced with a little help from the endorphin release of solitary long distance runs and its agency of insight tinged with well-being.

It was during this idyllic time that my paternal grandmother began experiencing some difficulty with swallowing. There was something foreboding about how my parents regarded this development that got my attention. My relationship to her was always profoundly close, very much on par with that of my mother. In short order, she was diagnosed with an essentially untreatable cancer and given a prognosis of death within the year. Already slightly built, she lost weight to the point of emaciation, required a tracheostomy to breathe, and experienced a precipitous decline.

Unable to speak, she would write short notes during our visits. Once, after my father left her hospital room for a moment, she scrawled on a pad and handed it to me, her eyes gesturing toward the door and shaking her head, which I took as her preference that it should stay between us. It said, "I hope I'm finished now." Our eyes locked and I said, "Me too," then stashed the note in my pocket. It remained our secret.

We visited again on the following day, and she was absolutely radiant. With bright, sparkling eyes, sitting up in bed, she smiled broadly as my dad and I entered the room. My hope soared as I thought that perhaps I was seeing a miracle. I would later come to understand that in a way, I was. The spirit, beyond human awareness, was gathering its remaining resources for one last great expression of love and joy, one last great projection of its holy self to simply say goodbye. We would take that image into our hearts, perhaps forever. Next day, she was gone.

My father and I always had trouble speaking with each other, especially as I moved through the teen years. We were just so very different, and those were the days of a great generational divide in the culture as well. Yet on the occasion of my grandmother's passing, a door opened, and we found a way. We were alone in the car immediately following her death when he began sharing spontaneously as I'd never heard before. Mostly he talked, and for a change, I really listened. As I recall, I was dumbfounded. Though he was a strict Catholic, he did not speak the language of the Church. Instead, he spoke from the apparent fruits of his contemplations, sharing an esoteric philosophy that extended well beyond the boundaries of the Faith. At the time, it struck me as a bit peculiar that my staunchly conservative, stoic father was speaking of a belief in multiple dimensions of experience, planes of existence, the infinite nature of life, and the role of death as a portal to something wondrous. He never let on what the source of these perceptions may have been, and I'd never seen any books around the house that would have led him to such notions. More, they seemed to have been born of a kind of tangible inner experience. He just seemed to know this stuff. Looking back, it is one of the great tragedies of our relationship that we never spoke of this again, but I believe he served as an early agent of my deepening curiosity about the nature of death and its role in the continuance of life.

My grandfather had left the making of funeral arrangements entirely to my dad, who, being the planner he was, had taken care of most of the details in advance. Together, he and I visited the Harland Funeral Home to attend to the few remaining matters.

Mr. Harland captured my attention from the first. In short order, he made us aware of how long he'd been in the business, how he'd seen pretty much everything, yet still had a passion for dignified funeral service. Because this was New York City, he told us, everything was unionized, jobs well defined. He was now a Director, but made it clear to us that he began his career as an Embalmer. He clearly maneuvered the conversation to make sure we knew that he was a man who had dirtied his hands in the interest of his craft. It was also clearly important to him that we should know he wasn't heartless, nor hardened by all these years with dirtied hands bearing witness to the seeming infinite ways humans come to die. There were situations over which he could still shed tears. I think his eyes actually moistened as he said this. He went on to say that my grandmother would be in the best of hands with a man named Billy who was experienced, skilled, and importantly to Mr. Harland, also fast.

Mr. Harland fascinated me, as did his work.

Billy did his job reasonably well given what he had to work with. My father had opted for a closed casket during calling hours, but the immediate family had a viewing. Mr. Harland had led us into the room by saying to my father, "Let's all go in. Mom looks great." Even at my tender age, I knew what to make of that. It was a setup, but probably a well-intentioned one. After all, Mr. Harland had a heart, even if my grandmother's body clearly lacked a soul.

I remembered how illumined she was that last time we were with her, but now, as hard as I looked, I could not find her. Perhaps this was helpful.

The following day we buried my grandmother in the midst of an impersonal ocean of headstones in one of those immense and anonymous New York City cemeteries. It was the first time I experienced leaving forever the body of someone who had been with me since the beginning of memory. It was the end of denial, the first real hint of the absolute finality that is death of the body along with its personality. So there and then, for my grandmother, I did mourn, and mourned deeply. I mourned the idea of moving forward on a planet absent of her forever, and for childhood gone, as finished and empty as her form now buried and earthbound. Even though an end, it was a beginning of something for us both.

Back at home in Connecticut, Mr. Harland and his invisible colleague Billy, along with the mysterious ways of their work, continued to cross my mind in the year or so that followed. I envied their proximity to something which held such fascination for me. I wanted to find a way into their world, to be one of death's people, to get my hands into it. I wanted an immersion and the familiarity it would bring. Even though I had officially committed to a Navy enlistment at the end of summer following high school, I was naively considering that perhaps funeral service should eventually become my life's work. My father knew an older man who was an embalmer for a local undertaker, and casually mentioned my interest to him. As the result of their conversation, it was suggested to me that I write him a letter.

Joe and I sat together one afternoon in an empty parlor of Trask Brothers Funeral Home. With my letter in his lap, looking at me over the top of his reading glasses, he broke the silence by simply saying, "Hell of a note you wrote here. I shared it with Pat and Rob Trask, and they want to meet you. They'll be along in a minute." He began to tell me how he got into the work as a young man in the 1930s, and how wakes used to take place in the family home. Because most people died there, they would embalm in the kitchen, and the wakes (particularly Irish) could go on for days, so thoroughness was essential especially during summer. He spoke in a matter-of-fact way about how they operated back then and how so much changed once services moved into the funeral homes. I began to feel as though I was being taken in trust, allowed to know some secret things and I warmed to it, asking questions to the extent I could.

Pat and Rob joined us, and after their introductions began peppering me with questions about the nature of my interest, presumably to determine if I was just morbidly curious or a serious player. Deciding I was the latter, they told me I had come to their attention at an interesting time. Prior to reading my letter, they had been lamenting how the embalming schools in New York and Boston were graduating people who had only a theoretical sense of the business. They would apply for two-year apprenticeships at funeral homes only to find they were ill-suited for the work. The Trasks thought perhaps the solution could be found in providing a one-year apprenticeship before attending school, then completing it after graduation. They were clear that what they were looking for was an all-around employee; one who could transition between doing removals, learning the fine points of embalming and layout, attending to wakes and funerals, meeting with families, along with washing cars and performing general housework. They were also okay with my Navy commitment. If things worked out, we'd pick up where we left off.

I was paired with Joe, who, as it turned out, had a reputation in the business for being among the best of embalmers, known for his ability to turn out a natural-looking body (a high compliment indeed). I would be learning from the best. We would be on call every other night and every other weekend—a system that made for up to 80 hour working weeks. Trask Brothers was a busy place. Our counterparts were John and Jerry. John, around Joe's age was very good as well, known as a thorough preservationist. Jerry, in his late twenties, was newly licensed and quite talented, drawing the best from both John and Joe.

I learned immediately that working with the dead and their survivors required great discretion, both regarding the ways of our work, and what we often came to know of those under our care. We also had our trade secrets which I honor to this day. Explicit descriptions of specific techniques may seem harmless in the moment, but when the person being informed experiences their own loss of a loved one, or recalls past loss, images will likely come to mind. No good can come of this. I also learned that respect and integrity were essential. When Joe first began teaching me, he was very clear, telling me, "Stevie, we work gently and quietly, as if this person is watching over us, because who's to say they're not?"

The dead feel different to the touch. Many assume this to be true, because there seems to be a natural aversion to it. So, for obvious reasons, in order to work in the field, it's the first thing to be overcome. We've all heard the term *cold* applied to bodies absent of life, but this is largely incorrect. Most of the objects we touch reflect the temperature of the environment, and this is the case with inert bodies. It's more a matter of what we expect, what experience has told us how a thing should feel. Like most of the observations surrounding all things dead, it's the recognition of something missing that our senses of sight and touch reveal. Repetition breeds familiarity, and even though the senses come to adapt to new expectations, the difference between the feel and sight of something charged with life and something absent of it will always be quite noticeable. Looks can sometimes deceive, but touch removes all doubt.

Oh, but the eyes. At times closed, but so often still open, the shades left up to varying degrees. Windows to the soul, it is said. Windows into the emptiness as well. They can be echoes—echoes of what was just seen in the moment when departing life suspended everything as it left, a minor chord of expression, something unresolved. Sometimes there was peace and relief, sometimes wonder and awe, sometimes shock and incomprehension.

Of course, our job was to remove that expression in favor of a resting one, allowing the veil of illusion to fall over those who would gather to honor the fallen and their kin. But as we worked, I would ponder this, silently asking them, "What did you see?" As I became more comfortable with Joe, as he gave me indications of his approval of my work and ways, I finally broached the subject with him.

"Joe, have you ever wondered about the eyes? Ever wondered about what they could possibly have seen just as it happened?"

"Stevie, I do. Every time. After 40 years of this I still wonder. How could I not? Personally, I think they see God." He paused a moment. "I think they see God, and maybe, depending on how they were when they were still alive, that can be either good news or not so good. But honestly, the more I look, the less I know. One thing is for sure—someday we'll all find out!"

"I thought it was just me. Thanks."

"Nah kid. We all think about that."

For the remainder of my brief apprenticeship with Trask Brothers, I wondered. I did so because the dead themselves left mostly questions and disappointingly few answers. Besides, I was told, funerals are not for those passed—they are for those who remain.

Attending to the dying during the following Navy years would encourage a different kind of wondering as I beheld the process of life departing its earthly frame of reference. Old Harland was right. No two deaths were ever the same. Sometimes it was a gentle release like Jim's, at other times a struggle to the final breath, sometimes the result of attempted resuscitation's violence, and others all the shades in between. But then it would be done, as irretrievably done as done could be. And each time I would consider what had just happened, what had become of the essence, the being that had only moments before, so clearly animated the now-still body before me.

Life is of course informed by experience, but I found it to be particularly so in the case of spending time with the dead and dying at such a young age. It set a foundation for virtually all my future spiritual exploration. I came to regard death as something holy and compelling, a continuation of creation itself. It became a familiar and omniscient teacher.

*   *   *

My mother told me she didn't fear dying of itself. Diagnosed during her 67th year with a metastatic cancer that had spread from bowel to liver, lungs, and brain, she seemed almost eerily reconciled to setting her life aside. But what she did fear was pain associated with dying.

"I don't want to be a baby," she told me.

"You won't be. I know this."

"How can you say that?"

"Because in all the times I've seen this kind of thing, no one has ever been a baby."

We had many late night, almost whispered phone conversations during her last year. Some had to do with mutual amends making; some were about repeatedly extracting a promise from me that I'd look after my father and troubled son, and still others were about her doubts of being worthy of entrance to heaven. But so often, it was about her being heard, which made sense because her life had not lent itself to that. She would speak about how she'd always felt directed toward servitude and compliance, the kind one allows begrudgingly from a deeply held notion that this is what is expected of a good girl raised in an immigrant Catholic home with an older brother. She seemed to have fallen under the spell of suffering as the way to attain heaven after living on a decidedly unheavenly earth, where a life of disappointment, self-perceived inadequacy, and subjugation were her lot. There was always a tone of grievance in her voice, the kind that comes from finally realizing the folly of all she thought she knew. Death's onset was teaching her these things, as both the need and ability to please others was fast and finally leaving her.

A few months before her death, I made a promise. I told her that when the time came for her to go, she would not be alone—I'd be with her. It seemed to settle her, and I was grateful for the thought that inspired it. I was also thankful for the experiences which allowed me to make that promise with such confidence.

I knew she was close. The numerous tumors in her liver had come to render it almost useless. In a twisted irony, this woman who had barely touched alcohol for her entire life was now jaundiced, and the accompanying rising ammonia levels in her brain had put her deep into an unending sleep. I'd spent the previous night in a recliner beside her hospice bed, waking about every 20 minutes to reach over and touch her hand so I'd know. Earlier in the evening, I'd whispered in her ear and told her whenever she wanted to let go would be fine—that her other children needed her too. Come the morning, I knew it would be her last.

My father arrived early in the day, and I told him her time was coming soon. We sat with her for a long while. He was to her right, hands folded in his lap as his eyes seemed to focus on some far away memory. I was to her left with one hand on hers, my other hand stroking her forehead. Abruptly, he stood up and told me he was going outside to smoke. I nodded and watched as he left the room.

Looking back to her, I remembered how we spoke on one particularly late night about her three dead children. She referred to them as "the kids," and said she felt they would all be reunited were she allowed to go to heaven. I wondered if she really believed this would be so, if I'd heard a question in her voice.

Two had passed just after birth, one just before; her last child gone by the time she was 32. She knew it would happen with every conception after me, and as strict Catholics, my parents were forbidden to practice any kind of birth control other than the rhythm method. These deaths occurred due to a blood incompatibility between her and my father, and subsequently between her and the children. It was during her pregnancy with me that she became sensitized. I survived without incident only because I was the first.

What I wanted to know, was how they could possibly have engaged in all the domains of a marital relationship at such a young age, knowing the outcome of conception would likely be death. Acknowledging my place as their child, I never asked either of them. But I gathered the answer was that they could not. Within the sacred confines of their marriage, they somehow decided in favor of their Faith, and in that final intimacy, condemned their marriage to death. And then there were four to mourn. My mother never told me how they grieved individually or as a couple other than some vague, almost absurd reference to "the Faith seeing us through." She never spoke about how they dealt with the enormity of what had happened, or if they ever regretted their decision.

What I can recall seeing for myself back then was a cordial, stoic, and distant couple, absent of the joy I saw with friends' parents. I observed significant disagreement between them only three times, and on each occasion, they didn't speak to each other for days, the loaded air viscous with tension. Then after all of these nearly unbearable incidents, they simply resumed with each other as if nothing had happened.

This mournful version of marriage, this elegy to which they had been delivered, could never have sustained the love giving, life producing expectations of their religion's definition of marital purpose. To me, it seemed doomed to wither away and decay into a life infused with guilt and shame and lack, a life to be endured and given over to melancholy, to grief unanswered.

In these, my mother's last moments of her earthly life, I was given to confront something that I'd never before considered: If it was possible that the sad, oppressive, and disappointing quality of her life as she perceived it, the crushing aggregate of loss and sacrifice, frustration and depression, all of the suppression and spiritual bypassing—if these toxicities were such that through some faculty of the mind or soul, she would have been able to summon forth this kind of death as a premeditated and gentle mercy—a surreptitious yet tender suicide. Did she, do we, have such power? Would "the Faith" have ever allowed such a thing?

My mother made a gentle noise, briefly inhaled, and left as sweetly as I'd ever seen anyone leave. It was the touch that told me. And I wondered. I wondered if she had waited for her husband to leave the room. I wondered if he knew as he left. Could it be that enduring couples can be complicit in spirit about these things? Maybe one last dance for these two; a last romantic thing. When he returned, I met him outside the room and told him she'd left us, but he responded as if he'd already known. It was something in his eyes. Yet even now, there was nothing for him to say.

Six or seven years had passed when I noticed my father had become elderly. Unsteady and frail, he became unable to walk more than 15 or 20 feet without stopping to catch his breath. This seemed to have happened suddenly, but perhaps it was my noticing that was sudden. It was like that between us.

He had developed chronic, severe lung disease, the result of a lifelong smoking habit, an addiction he'd been unable to overcome. Breath was being progressively denied him. I can't think of anything more frightening than the inability to move enough air. There had been several hospitalizations, each more involved than the one before, each carrying more suffering and uncertainty. And each time he would count the days before he could return home to smoke more cigarettes, sometimes attempting to joke about this in order to mitigate his shame. For me, listening to that was an opportunity to practice compassion and tolerance and nonjudgement. I was often unsuccessful with these things. Our relationship was flawed and difficult, loaded with long standing mutual disappointment, but knowing we were reaching our end moved me to at least try. His approaching death was encouraging me to attempt to live in a better way.

It was nearly 13 years after my mother's passing when my father's time finally came—long years he had missed her terribly, years he had not removed the wedding ring from his left hand. I think there were conversations, though he was too reserved and private to freely admit it. I'd never have asked, but I really do think he spoke to her. His later days were marked by extreme solitude. He had no relationships to speak of, so other than my weekly visits, he would spend his time as alone as one could imagine. He said he preferred this. He demonstrated his preference for this. I believed him.

I'd walk into his place and we'd offer each other the same mutual greeting as the time before and the time before that. We'd sit together and honor my mother—me by fulfilling the promise I made to her that I'd look after him, and him by wearing that ring as if she'd never left. And while our predictable and mundane conversations ran on as a matter of ritual, the things I really wanted to know about remained tucked away, carefully stowed forever. I'd wonder if beneath the weight of his stoicism, he'd felt any of it: The deaths of three infant children, the sorrowful marriage, the disappointments, the way things turned out. All I could have said with absolute confidence about him was that he wished to be alone.

Dad's death was quite unlike my mother's. My primary role in his was to help him prepare. It was during his final hospital stay when the nurse approached as I left one evening and proposed I should talk with my father. I knew about what. The nurse was apparently unaware that my father and I were not given to speaking of such things, that there was an element of absurdity to the suggestion.

He and I did speak, and it went something like this:

"I need to talk to you about how this is going."

"Oh?"

"This thing can't be fixed and it's not going to get any better. We have to shift gears, Dad."

"Go on."

"We have to shift from treatment to comfort. It's time."

"Seems pretty serious." His tone seemed patronizing.

"I've asked hospice to send someone in to chat with us. She'll be here tomorrow."

"Hospice! It's come to that?"

"It has. I'm sorry Dad, but you need to know where things stand."

At this point he paused, staring past me, being with it for a long moment. After a time, his gaze returned to me.

"I want it fast and I want it painless." It sounded like an instruction.

"Painless I will promise you. Fast is between you and God."

A few more minutes passed. Then he told me I had been a

good son. This was enough for us, for me. It is the inheritance I've thought of the most since then.

I sat with him through his last night. Now unconscious, his breathing was agonal, each respiration carrying the potential of being his last. One of my hands rested atop his, a gesture that neither of us would have allowed were he still conscious. It was getting late, and I knew the following day would require more from me than a sleepless night would allow. I had to leave him, but couldn't. I remembered my time as a young man, idealistically convinced no one should die alone, keeping watch with relative strangers as they folded in. Why them and not my father? Why my mother but not my father? Wasn't it my duty to see him off as well? What of the promise I'd made to Mom that I would look after him? It had always been just us three.

My dearest one was with her family out of state, so I called her because I needed her to tell me, even though to ask would have been unfair. Grace itself answered as we spoke. Without me having to ask, she reminded me of how much he preferred being alone, how it had been his way, and suggested that maybe his preference meant more than my expectation—that maybe this was something he needed to do alone. I remembered him leaving my mother, going outside when her time had come. I always wondered what he thought as he stood out there alone, smoking. Perhaps he and I were now complicit as I suspected they may have been. Permission given, I said my simple goodbye and then left him with all of what was his to do.

I took the long way home and drove slowly just like he always did, drove slowly as an homage, drove slowly to remember. I spoke to him in the quiet of my car and told him many things—some that couldn't wait any longer, words too late from my lips. I told him how he was an enigma to me, his personality so utterly odd it was impossible to penetrate. I told him he did well with this because his defense had been impenetrable, just as he wanted it to be. Both of us only children, I understood his need for this. I also pointed out to him it was hard to be enigmatic as he lay dying—it's the great and absolute leveler of vulnerability's playing fields.

Arriving home, I sat out for a while on that warm, close, summer night as the sounds of insect life in the surrounding trees lulled me into memory, stringing along our old story on the hum and the chirp and the stitch, heard only in perfect, still air. I was looking for the ending of that story. How futile and unwise of me to think such a thing.

I looked at my hands and saw his; the shape of my fingers and nails, their structure, their persistent evidence of lineage. I noticed how the backs of these old hands of mine were beginning to take on the same crepey etch of the skin, though on my palms I noticed also the slightly rougher finish of periodic manual labor absent from his. My hands are a continuing of him, and so it seems of our story. Their two sides, the similarities and differences, will remind me of him as long as I am given to live or able to remember. When a nurse called me at 4:30 next morning to advise me of my father's passing, it was my hands I looked to first as a way of centering, of turning the final page on our penultimate chapter.

* * *

Often, we're not alone with the dying. Sometimes there is the power of *we*.

Kenny had called me during the late afternoon. Our weekly Men's Spirituality Discussion Group was to meet that evening. He rarely missed. A brittle diabetic, he suffered from a chronic infection in one of his feet. Typically, only being hospitalized with that would cause him to miss one of our gatherings. They were as important to him as his attendance was to us. He was calling to say he felt exhausted and weak—that he was having trouble with swallowing and hadn't eaten in days. I could hear the concern and weakness in his voice and prayed he could not hear the dread in mine. Of course, my grandmother's condition came to mind…as well as the foreboding.

The following week found us holding our meeting in his cramped hospital room. I had spoken with Kenny's wife earlier. She said he was found to be "loaded" with tumors; that he'd be told by the doctors the next day when his entire family could be there. Our topic that night was about how much our group's discussions had meant to each of us, and the kinds of things they had taught us. I've come to believe that even life confined to the human domain is far too expansive for us to be denied an intrinsic sense of its coming end, so I think he instinctively knew the score that night as he voiced his thoughts with a quiet courage and freedom only the dying can know.

A few weeks later we met again, this time in his hospice room. Kenny was awake for most of our time together. He said beautiful things to us, and we to him. We did not choose a topic our final night. It chose us. Our topic for the evening was love, in retrospect the only one we'd ever had, and I think maybe we each heard something that made it all okay. We heard him call us all his good friends as we said goodbye. He fell asleep as we all left.

Next morning, his family gathered around as he laid unconscious. His mother was there along with Sue, his wife, and Krista, his daughter, and in the true spirit of hospice care, his dog was with him too, taking his station at the foot of the bed. His brother and sister-in-law were driving the 200 miles from their home, having been summoned earlier that morning. Although not related to Kenny, I was there as well representing his other, chosen family, those who had shared his last lucid moments the night before. He and I had spent quite a bit of time together over many years, and even though all agreed I belonged, I mostly kept a respectful, peripheral position in the room.

Before too long, Sasha, a middle-aged woman with long, gray hair and dressed in bohemian fashion wearing an official ID badge, came into the room carrying a guitar case along with a sweet and gentle disposition. She asked if we'd like her to play some music. We looked at each other smiling because there were few things other than his family that Kenny loved more than music. Although he couldn't carry a tune in a bucket, he had what could be considered an encyclopedic knowledge of, and profound appreciation for, meticulously well played, seriously loud music. Although Sasha could not provide much in the way of volume, she had walked into a most appreciative audience. Opening her guitar case with a well-practiced movement, she extracted her instrument and asked what kind of music Kenny liked. His wife, daughter, and I all replied at the same time: "Blues," we said. And so it went. Though now completely unresponsive, he'd have been quite okay with her playing and singing. She remained for about an hour, and it really did wonders for the room.

His wife and daughter knew he was dying, knew this with certainty, but Mom kept a more hopeful vigil. I really believe she thought there was a chance he would somehow survive. How else could a mother reconcile this? She had just turned 90, and in the mild confusion of her age, understanding such an out-of-time passing as this was just beyond any reasonable expectation. To me, she seemed locked in and distant, perfectly unavailable to this particular mother-and-son drama. She appeared to be dreaming of other times; perhaps staring at her boy through a kitchen window, forever young and full of endless possibility, running across summer lawns, playing with his dog, or building snowmen with his brother. Maybe too, she dreamed of the time when she carried him within, feeling the closeness of his movements and kicks, their sharing of life's rhythms and cycles, her anticipation of what he would be like and how they might be with each other, an intimacy well beyond the scope of any words that could ever be spoken. It is one thing to know someone, but to have carried them in pregnancy is a sacrament. His very life had come out of her. Surely, he would somehow awaken and return. For him to be dying seemed impossible. Mothers grieve impossibly.

There came a subtle shift in the collective mood of the room, as if it was time for a kind of movement. Kenny's wife and daughter stood and one of them mentioned they should go outside to smoke. My own available time was running short, and I began to think I should leave soon as well. His mother remained seated in a large chair fairly close to her son. I walked his wife and daughter out and into the hallway where I let them know I'd likely be leaving soon, and said my goodbyes. As I watched them walk down the hall, I saw Kenny's brother Paul and sister-in-law Linda come off the elevator. I greeted them as they approached, and told them where things stood.

"It's good you're here," I said. "He's so very close."

They both looked past me into the room. "See you soon," I added, and looked one last time at what remained of my friend before leaving. My goodbye from the night before would suffice.

A few days later I walked into the wake. I passed Kenny's photo atop the box containing his ashes, made my way to the family and hugged them all. I spoke briefly with Sue and Krista, then to Paul and Linda. Paul told me he wanted a word when we could get away for a moment. I went to his mother next and sat beside her. She smiled and immediately thanked me for being there "on the day my boy died," then told me how much Kenny thought of our friendship. I waited a moment, took her hand in mine, and as our eyes met, told her, "I'm sorry you've lost your baby." She never replied, but only glanced back toward the box and the photo.

I stayed for the entirety of the wake. Mostly, I chatted with old friends and marveled at how the conversation at such gatherings avoids any substantive discussion of death itself. Stories about the deceased (now the proper term for Kenny) flowed freely, and many really were quite funny. More than a few folks remarked that because he was only 60 years old, this somehow did not constitute a "full" life. I kept to myself on this because I have no way of knowing such a thing. Seemed pretty full to me.

I noticed Paul sitting alone and staring at his brother's container as the crowd began to thin. I sat next to him and gave him a gentle elbow that startled him out of his reverie.

"Oh hey!" he said, smiling. "Thanks for waking me up."

"So, brother Paul," I said. "Tell me what happened after I left you."

He turned more toward me in his seat. "How did you know he was so close to dying?"

I replied that I'd been privileged to see this many times before—that he'd been unconscious since the previous night, had never come out of that, and, for the entire time we were with him on the morning he died, his breathing had become agonal. I asked why he wanted to know.

He shook his head slowly, and glanced again toward his brother's remains.

"Linda and I walked in and said hi to Mom for a minute. Then I got on the side of the bed he was more turned toward, and Linda was across from me. I noticed that weird breathing you mentioned. All I said was his name and told him I was there."

He shook his head again, then continued: "It wasn't a minute went by, and he opened his eyes wide, then closed them, then opened them again and looked right at me. Looked right at me!" Paul paused a moment. "And then he took this one great big last breath."

"Can't say for sure, but it sounds to me like he might just have waited for you," I said.

"But how? How does that happen?"

I shrugged. "Life is way bigger than we are, brother Paul."

We spoke for a time about Kenny; how it had seemed to me that he and Paul were two very different men, yet drawn so close by the love inherent in family. There was a parallel in our respective relationships in that Kenny and I were two very different men as well, yet drawn close in a fellowship of common experience, a different kind of family. And as we spoke, we found this brother of ours had bestowed on each of us a mystical moment during the process of his dying. It was a moment that transcended any perceived differences of personality or circumstance or anything of a temporal nature.

For Paul, it was this unexplainable yet pretty obvious waiting, an imparting of something of value which was still being revealed to him, a thing he was still trying to understand, something in that last look. For me, it was a moment just he and I had shared the night before his death during his final hours of earthly awareness—something he saw, or, more correctly, something in the way of a vision. Kenny had found a way to teach us both. Death was the portal to this teaching, and in the unique community which formed around his passing, it also managed to show us the power of a unified *we* that lies at our very center.

There are those among us who have had much more time and immersion with death and those who are dying than I. From my travels through this world which lies at the cusp of the next, the hospice nurses come to mind. I don't think it unreasonable to characterize them as comforters and way showers, as angels. They stand in the thin place—their feet kindly planted here, but with an awareness extending beyond. I believe their placement in this work inherently falls in the realm of a calling. How else could it be? Is there anything nobler than this? Typically, they are seasoned nurses who previously functioned at a high level in the acute-care world, but for an infinite variety of reasons were drawn to this most fundamental place. I knew one of them particularly well.

When we first met, she was an Intensive Care Unit Nurse, talented and incredibly capable. There are those who are born for their work, and she was one. At that time, I worked in the clinical laboratory and blood bank, so our paths crossed often. We were on the night shift then, and as in most hospitals there was a great deal of comradery among the staff of the various departments. In a way, it was like family.

On one particular night, I was passing through the unit, and noticed her in a darkened room absent of the usual level of technology. She was leaning in close, whispering into the ear of a seemingly unconscious, dying woman, one arm draped around the top of the pillow. I saw a genuine humanity and compassion, an intimacy and peace strikingly odd in this place of dramatic and sometimes violent interventions. There was a palpable sense that something quietly dignified and sacred was transpiring. I recalled sitting with Jim and the others nearly 20 years before at the Naval Hospital.

She and I spoke about it on the following night shift in the wee hours, across a table in the breakroom of the ICU. I always found the general weariness at such a time of day lends a vulnerability to the moment, a willingness to go to the heart of things. I told her I wanted to know more about what I'd observed, what an arresting and moving scene it had been. And yet, oddly, there didn't seem to be any one question that was coming to mind.

"Can you tell me about what happened?" I finally asked.

"Yeah," she said. "It doesn't happen like that often around here. It was a slow night otherwise, so I was able to get her cleaned up and spend some time after we discontinued everything. She was essentially in full body failure, you know?"

"I remember the lab numbers," I replied. "Pretty much screwed."

"It's nice to have some quiet time with them," she offered, smiling a little.

"So, what were you saying to her?"

"I think they're often reluctant to leave. They fight what's happening. In her case, she had a huge family who all lived far away, and Mamas worry about things…makes them want to hang on. They need to know everything will be okay, so we give good drugs to slow the brain down, but they need more than that. I just told her it was okay to let go. She was religious, so I said the family and she were all in God's hands and everybody would be fine. I told her love can't die, so she could take that with her."

"That's it?"

"Pretty much. Isn't that what it all boils down to? I mean, after all this clinical stuff has run its course, it just needs to be okay."

"I've never seen something like that on the ICU. That was beautiful."

"I do it whenever the work allows," she said. "I think when I'm older and I can't keep up with this anymore, I'm gonna do Hospice care. It just seems right."

I told her of my time at the Naval Hospital, and how I felt it so important to keep company with those who were at the end of their time.

"It just never occurred to me that I should have said anything," I told her.

"We have five senses, and hearing still works well until the end so I think it's good to make use of that." She leaned across the table toward me. "But still, it's sweet how you took the time to be with them. To tell you the truth," she confided, "I did that too when I was a nursing student."

"I can only hope they somehow knew," I said.

"How couldn't they?" she asked.

Around 15 years later, matters of family and her health strongly suggested she should make a change. So, after health care had fully become managed care, and everything that happened within the confines of the hospital began to sour and break her heart, she escaped to one of the few places where true compassion remained—where the ratio of paper work to patient work retained its correct proportion. It was as if everything she had ever done as a nurse until then led her to care for the dying. Callings are like that.

* * *

It seems to me that I should expect some change in the perception of death's ways after a lifetime of goodbyes, but what can be seen of it has remained pretty simple all along. Through the biological circumstances of disease or some form of trauma, either suddenly or gradually the body is no longer able to support being animated, so it permanently collapses. It is a setting aside, a leaving behind, and ultimately done with a kind of sigh. For some time now, it has not impressed me as an ending. What has changed over time are my perceptions about the intangible something which would suddenly be absent beneath my touch. These days, I think perhaps a dreamer simply awakens and leaves behind the dreamed world, the dreamed body, the dreamed mind, the dreamed personality, much as any of us awaken from our sleeping dreams. Left behind are the fellow-dreamed who gather beside the casket to behold what remains as absent and vacant and un-whole. Something ancient deep within them maybe even begins to remember. While the conversation at such gatherings is usually geared to times remembered and avoidance of the obvious, private thoughts will often stray toward the existential.

I've wondered if it is true that life proceeds along a timeless continuum and our appearances on earth occur as prolonged cosmic days. If so, I've written the last several thousand words concerned with the sun setting on those days. But what of sunrise?

I could only see the very top of the skull, positioned as it was in the birth canal. It was stuck there, and I sensed the physician was becoming concerned. Though calm and measured, she was beginning to consider alternative approaches to resolve the problem.

We were in a birthing room, meant to be more like a bedroom than a delivery room—a less clinical atmosphere. The year was 1981, early in the American application of Lamaze as a birthing technique. I had earned my "right" to be in the room by attending classes with my wife which would allow us to function as part of the team bringing our child into the world. It made good sense. Our fathers had been relegated to the waiting room where they paced and smoked and worried, while our mothers were often anesthetized and operated upon.

Finally, the doctor made her call.

"I think we need to go to the delivery room," she said. "The table there is harder than the bed, and the angle will help too. I know you both want to have your baby here, but I really think it would be better to move now."

There was a concerned tone in her voice, and she leaned on the word *now*. We moved.

There was a sudden, seemingly unending surge of blood-tinged fluid as his body twisted through, freed of its confinement at last. At a moment like this, memory can replay almost in still frames, slower than slow motion, every minute detail seared in and recalled perfectly. At a moment like this, memory is infallible.

His body was like glistened porcelain, unanimated and unoccupied. Recalling past experiences, I looked away, terrified, maybe even horrified, certainly overwhelmed. It was as if the air pressure in the room had changed, weighted and loaded with a collective disquiet. A nurse began verbalizing health assessment scores which were poor.

But then the sounds of the room muffled and faded into something like a distant echo, and a voiceless, wordless thought came—my first exposure to such a thing. It compelled me to look as surely as if two hands had grasped my head. I saw the pale, empty, bloody-wet mannequin that was his body, come into its being with a simple twitch. I remember this as something of the eternal and holy, the power behind it unspeakable, as if an entire universe had just come into existence. There was breath, then color and movement and a healthy wail of vehement protest—the sun rising. I held him first.

A little more than two years later, came our daughter. Now we were seasoned, labor went more smoothly, and I was prepared for a second coming similar to the first. Once again, I thought, I would have the privilege of bearing witness to a blossoming of human form. Through all the rapidly progressing stages of labor, anticipation built. Now as she crowned, I peered in, and in no uncertain terms, I knew that life had already taken up its body. She spun into the outer world present and animated, beautiful and perfect from the start. It had been hers to experience. There was no vehement protest, and I had the sense she was okay with being here. I cut her umbilical cord, a ritual denied during the concern and duress of her brother's birth, and placed her blanketed body on her mother's belly.

I suppose this matter of birthing really is analogous to the sunrise in that no two are ever the same, nor are the days that follow. Sometimes there is the wonder of a thousand illumined colors playing off a few clouds splashed across a horizon, the vision changing by the moment. At other times the clouds are thick and dark, leaving light's arrival somewhat ambiguous. The days that follow a rising sun as it arcs across the sky have never been the same for anyone—each day, each moment for that matter, its very own world loaded with infinite possibility. What dreams might come this day?

And as sunset approaches, we will often reflect on the waning day, trying to make some sense of what we think has happened.

Perhaps this is not as reliable as we've been led to believe, as fewer things make much sense at all. With age we notice as the passage of time seems to compress, finally revealing its illusion as the days appear to move by more quickly, and we begin to understand it has been both our servant and master. Time is coming to pass beyond time. Time's up. Time flies. Time and again. Time to go. And the sun sets. What kinds of dreams might come near our day's end? For me, such a dream as this, conjured out of deep missing and a measure of regret:

The first thing is to climb the steep berm of the dune, following the sounds from the surf beyond. At the top, it's not unusual for those who've never been here, or who, like me don't come often, to stop and pause as one might when entering a church sanctuary. From here I can see the entire crescent of the beach: the Atlantic, the sand, the grasses, the hook of the point a mile distant. Past that is an inlet which leads to the bay sheltered behind this peninsula of beach and grasses. The cloudless sky is cerulean, and the sun is directly overhead as it pours warmth, softening the chill of a stiff breeze blowing off the water. I descend to the beach and spot him right away, standing knee deep in the surf, hands in the pockets of his rolled up white jeans. Older now and intrinsically wise, he glances back knowing I'm now here, and even though it's been some time, he doesn't seem too exuberant at the sight of me. I think he may be smiling, though, as he turns back toward the endless horizon of the ocean to fill the time as I make my way.

We somehow agreed to meet here, purposefully avoiding anywhere we may have already been together. It seemed important to start with someplace new and apart from what was before. Memories can so distract us from the matter at hand, whatever that may prove to be. As we made our plans to meet, I had the sense that we'd been called by a common voice that remained between us and commanded our absolute trust.

I feel my breath becoming shallow with a quickening pulse, and my head feels a bit light. Understandable given our past. In circumstances such as these, identity can become fluid, and the one we seem to be with can resemble another. When is a son no longer a son, or a brother never known, a brother? Is it when one of us is still traveling in time, and the other has been freed? The distance between us closes slowly given the sand, the effort it adds to the walk, and the way my body is feeling. He is but a stone's throw away now, yet it feels as though it could take the rest of the day to reach him. Finally, I'm standing at the edge of the dry sand, while he remains in the shallow surf.

"Pops," he calls me, turning fully toward me at last and smiling warmly.

"Little brother," I call him, as I start to remove my sandals to join him in the water.

He holds up a hand. "How about you stay dry for now?"

I nod. We turn toward the far end of the beach and begin walking, he in the backwash of the waves, me on the sand. I find myself wondering what will happen when we reach the end at the inlet.

There are some others here, a scattered few, really. For such a perfect summer's day, I'd have expected more. I notice they are mostly women with a few children running about, and I sense they are familiar to me, though I can't imagine why. I choose to ignore them for now and focus on him.

I don't know where to begin. So much time has passed, so many thoughts and remembrances and of course the endless questions, but somebody needs to start. I have the distinct impression this falls to me.

"I've been daydreaming a lot about a road trip lately. Just you and me. Heading west to fuck knows where…driving until we run out of America, then heading north or south. I'd think a few thousand miles together might actually be good for us."

He nods his head as if he somehow already knew and smiles more broadly now. "Yeah," *he says.* "Wouldn't that be the shit?"

His eyes have changed. It's what I've noticed first. Even as he squints under the midday sun, I can see it. There was a time long ago when they had a dreadful weight, when they were opaque with anxiety and anger and mistrust, when it was like the light could neither enter nor escape, when he was feral and lived only for the next, for the next, for the next. But now they are placid, at rest for once, transparent and welcoming and transcendent of all that has passed between us. Perhaps forgiving eyes. Yes. Please let them be that.

"I've always felt I failed you, brother. In such fundamental ways. I think you know of my regret. To just say, 'I'm sorry' strikes me as an insult to you."

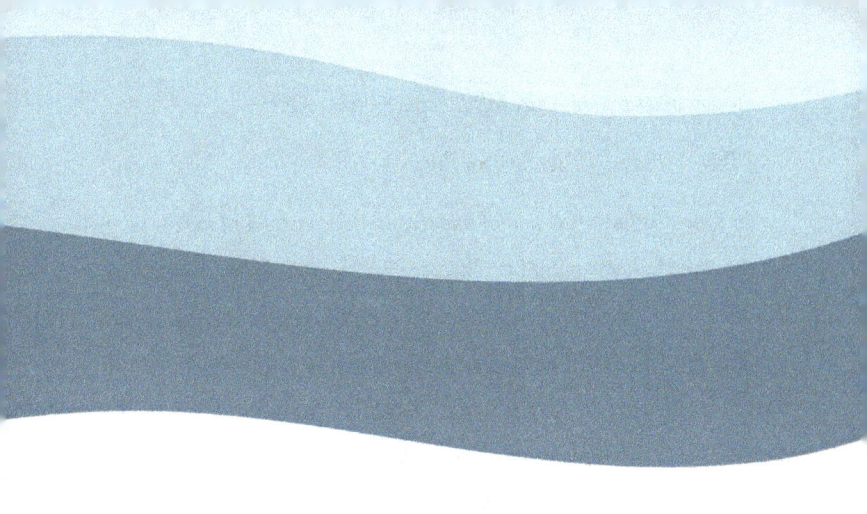

He regards me kindly, tilting his head a bit.

"Pop, this can't be about apologies. It's gotta start with the step after that. We've both been crucified. Enough." He glances down at the water for a moment, then back toward me. "Enough," he says once more. "You walked your long road. You know better now. I know you do." He stops and turns toward me. "Let me show you something."

The wind continues to blow, the water shimmers sunlight in the way that always makes me think of souls twinkling, the waves keep washing in, and I hear those children at play behind me. But he is still. Not just still as in not moving. Still as in a photographic image. I'm drawn to his soft, finely aged eyes. They seem to be the only part of him that has any kind of movement.

Absent of speech, his voice fills the space within me.

"There," it says. "Better now for this."

In time it is but a fraction of one second that passes, but here is all of what I come to know within it: There is one. Not two. It has always been this since before the before. In it is every thought, every feeling, every word that ever passed between us, but now known by us both as the other, because there is…only one. Everything said or thought or felt in the dream of two, now known as a complete and single reality. No more secrets. The two are gone. There is a kind of pause and we settle. The fraction of a second then ends. Time again. Two again. And now I know the full and complete effect of absolutely everything ever thought or said between or about us.

One could think this would be a problem, but it's not. It seems we have traveled beyond any judgment or hurt or resentment or even thoughts. We have traveled to simple yet pure knowing. Here, we find it all belonged, that it was all perfect. All the objects have been left at the altar—offered, cleansed, and released; their high purpose understood. Only the love remains.

Back now in the finite here of the beach, I feel compelled to go to him. Resistance is futile. I step into the surf, and the last thing I see of him are his eyes, happy and at peace. Without another word passed, he's gone. I spin around, searching, though I know what I've done. It's all gone quiet. And along the beach, the women and children are all photograph-still.

There was a lifetime of preparation for this one. It's been ten years now and honestly, I'm still not quite right about it. There's a difference between acceptance and being quite right. After this much time, I'm beginning to think it never will be, for it counts as the singular most devastating and dreadful thing I have ever known, an eruption of grief and longing that has eclipsed all others, a grief so profound it gives pause to the desire for life to continue. The arc of the sun across my boy's day was marked by a great measure of joy and beauty during its morning, but then darkness gathered around noon and descended with great authority. In retrospect, he'd seemed ambivalent about this life even as he came to it.

His was a life that gave me pause to wonder if there are those among us who are not long for this world. Not to suggest his appearance here was some cosmic accident, but clues were left along the way to suggest it wouldn't be old age that would lead him off.

At the very end, what did lead him off after 28 years was the quite intentional act of hanging himself in his bedroom closet. This means his death was due to choking, a lack of air, not something that happened instantly or comfortably or peacefully. I think it took great discipline and dedication to accomplish this. It took a lifetime of practice. I believe he found a way to tell the world, in this final act on earth, how unspeakable his reality had become. There were simply no more words to say to a world that could not hear.

News of his death came to me during a phone call with a police officer. I recall his kind patience with a grieving father whose utter shock could barely allow thought or speech. He sounded young, maybe even younger than my boy, and he kept telling me how sorry he was. I told him to tell me everything and he did. I asked about a note. None was found. There was nothing left to ask or say. My first conversation as a father whose son died had ended.

I kept telling myself he was finally at peace, that his nightmare was now over. I told myself this as my heart was disintegrating from the way I imagined he looked as it happened. And yet even as I kept envisioning that horrific sight in his bedroom closet, a vision that would not soon leave, my hands could still remember the warm, soft feel of him the first time I held his body and stroked the soft skin of his perfect cheek only moments after I had seen life come to him. It is that feel which haunts me still and echoes in my senses.

Despite the extremity of his demonstration, I'm still not convinced he wanted to die. Those who have survived their attempted suicide are generally clear about what their intentions had been. What they wanted was for the pain to end. In his case, the pain simmered for half of his life, repeatedly stirred and stoked and added to. Ultimately, the horror of his pain had simply matched his end. By the time he lost his grandmother, my mother, at the age of 18, he'd already experienced sexual, emotional, and psychological assault. For him, she had been a refuge, one of very few islands of respite and peace, of God's own love. It became time for him to set sail for other islands.

A little over six months after my mother passed, I received a call from his mom at around 4:00 in the morning. She told me our son had been stabbed during an altercation in a crack house. His liver had been lacerated, and as we spoke, they were getting him ready for surgery. This was fairly early in his addicted life, so we had not yet become accustomed to such things. Returning to sleep would not be likely. I made my way to the hospital later that morning after the surgery was done. Meaningful conversation proved impossible. All I could do was sit with him and weep. When conscious, he acted as if I was his burden.

I returned the following day. It was then I knew.

As part of his postoperative pain management, he was given a Patient Controlled Analgesia device. This computerized intravenous pump allows the patient to deliver a dose of opioid medication with the push of a button, though only within preset limits. It also records the number of times the button is pushed, allowing the staff to assess the efficacy of dosing and detect signs of dependency. One can clearly see how this would increase the nurse's efficiency.

I didn't have a good feeling about this. We spoke for a while, and he seemed more agreeable than he had been the day before. He was improving clinically, so they planned to discharge him soon. He talked lovingly about "the button" and how much he'd miss it. Then I watched as he hit the switch. His head tilted back into the pillow, and a look of utter bliss and peace and contentment came over his very being. In that one miraculous moment, everything changed. His pain and all that was or had ever been wrong with his life fled, and I watched as the wonder of it overwhelmed him. That look was unmistakable. I knew he had found his Answer. Years later he told me that he went from the front door of the hospital to the heroin dealer. Everything changed.

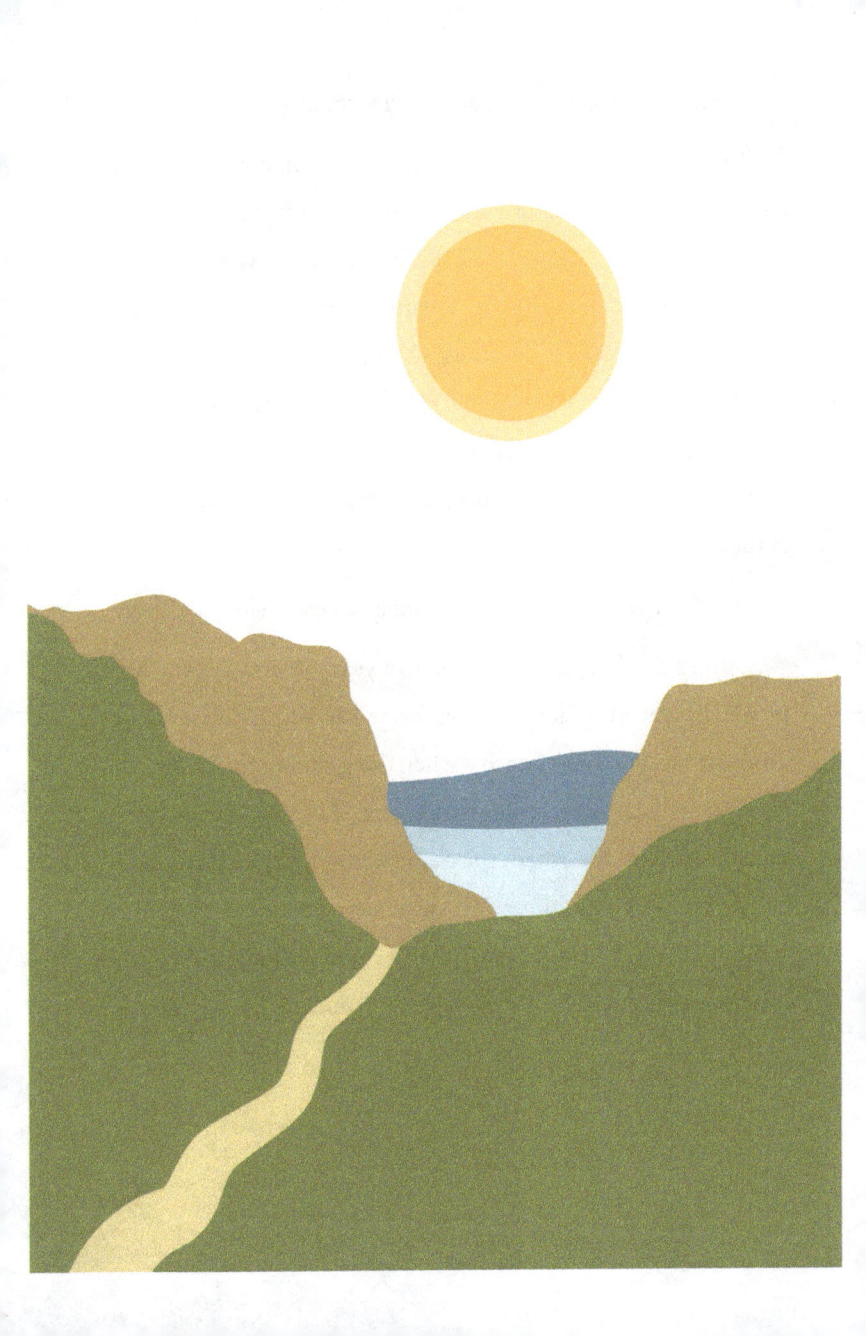

It went on for ten more years. Until it could go on no further.

There is little purpose in documenting the many waypoints of an addicted, deeply disturbed and corrupted life. Suffice to say it was extreme and it was horrific. Its ending, its movement toward something kinder and gentler, regardless of method, could have only arrived as a welcomed release. It had come to that. The unique problem for those of us who were there from its very beginning was in the futile attempt to reconcile the life we once held in our arms, its beauty and perfect innocence, with what was now laid before us in the casket.

Those who remain must find something to hold...in order to let go.

During the late spring of his 13th year, he and I went on a three-day canoe trip down the Delaware River with his Boy Scout Troop. It was not long after this when things began to change, so it remains my final sweet memory of many. Though there was much time shared with the others, the canoe was our very own place, and being there was everything. We switched positions at every stop, and I preferred the rear because then I could see him, and as I still can now: young and healthy, happy and contented, funny and yet strangely wise. We followed the river's gentle flow past beavers and otters, nesting bald eagles and stoic blue herons, while fleets of muskies and carp swam by just beneath the surface, easily seen through the pristine water. I like to think we could have remained on that river forever. I like to think we have.

Now, in this other time, in this other life, I can go there still. Time and the river have mercifully settled me, and granted the gift of noticing even the slightest whisper. On some warm late spring day, a breeze may blow, my head may turn to hear his voice spoken on that breeze, and something is kindly forgiven, an older, wiser way now known better to me—in a perfect canoe, on a gentle river, beyond just one more bend.

> We beached our beautiful canoe
> on a sandy shore beside the river
> just past a fine rapid run
> and made a good camp
> at the edge of the flood plain forest
> with a fire we made from friction

and dry things
no cheating.
We ate well and drank cleanly
as dusk fell-in
and all around was good quiet and blue light
and our voices which never rose above a whisper.
Never had to…so quiet.
Sleep came right there
beside the fire
and in the morning the light was golden amber
and the mist was rising thick from the river
and he was missing.
I made my way to the river's edge
to where the beautiful canoe had been.
And looking down-river I saw him fading
dissolving
into the mist
rounding a forever bend.
I called but no sound came.
No sound could.
All in a dream.

* * *

I've always been searching for something eternal and unchanging, something in the way of freedom and release from the sheer weight of the human experience. I'm hardly unique in this. As with so many of us, I've tended to look beyond myself and out into the world for such things. I've tried many of the usual methods to reconcile this relentless seeking, and some have led me nearly to the brink of my own mortality. Clearly this has been a mistake, for the world is made only of the shifting and changing, at best mere shadows of the eternal. Death, as well as a few other things, has been my good and steadfast teacher in this regard—something tangible and unambiguous to tell me that I am, we are, something more than a body, a personality, and that perhaps just beyond these things lies our wisdom and holiness, our truth.

The eyes of the dead and dying that have so fascinated me held at least part of the answer, for these were eyes that had shifted from sight to vision—what eyes look like when they no longer see the world but gaze inward, and so often for the first time. Those who experience death of the body as a more prolonged affair, those I've joined as they sat at this farthest edge of time before the no-time, tend to show little apparent fear in these moments when they are at their closest. It seems to be one of the great illusions to dissolve, a truth always known deep beneath the mesmerized life just lived—the kind of truth most clearly seen at a time like this when there is little need for illusions designed to protect us.

As they look about, the eyes of the dying see a new world, perhaps an in-between world. Sometimes this is reflected in a mild confusion, a befuddlement. If able, they will say strange, seemingly nonsensical things as they attempt to put in earthly terms something which is not.

I was with Kenny in his hospice room waiting for the others to arrive for our last gathering. We were having some light conversation when he seemed to notice something in my general direction, doing a double take. His eyes blinked repeatedly, he shook his head slightly a few times, and his mouth opened a little as if in wonder. I asked if there was anything wrong, if he was okay. Still looking in my direction, he let out a long, slow, "Whoa." A moment passed, and then a drawn out, "Wow." He settled for a moment and I asked with a grin if he saw something good. He just held up one hand and gently shook his head. This spoke volumes. I sensed I was in the company of one who stood at the garden gate holding the handle, first glimpsing the sweetly illuminated far country just beyond. This was not something that struck me as worthy of mourning. All I could think was, "Move on, dear brother! Go now and think of us as you do!"

Death as we know it is observed by us through the filter of all we've been shown from those who came before us, the culture in which we've been raised. Our suffering, our mourning, our agonizing grief is rooted in this context. We have learned well and deeply it is something to dread, loathe, and avoid at all cost even though it is utterly inevitable. It has become a horrible and terrible thing. It has become this because despite all our spiritual seeking through rituals and meditations and even drug induced shamanistic ceremonies, our ideas of life remain confined to what the senses will allow. We celebrate birth and grieve death based on the mistaken notion that this is all there is. Our idea of the eternal is mostly theoretical and therefore insufficient to soothe us. To live the life of a mystic seems counter-intuitive and suggests too much discipline of thought for most, but this is what would seem to be required of someone wishing to die beautifully. Those blessed with the experience of near death seem always to acquire the mystical view.

Of course, death as experienced by those dying appears to be another matter entirely. Although it could be dictated to some extent by the spiritual orientation of the life just lived, I've come to believe that when our time arrives, we will be given what we need as always, peace will prevail, and the world will simply dissolve before us, our dream here set aside as we awaken to what follows. It may be that we've been asleep all along, asleep to the truth of ourselves.

There is an often-observed phenomenon that seems to gather around or from within those departing as the time of their awakening approaches. It was my grandmother who first showed me this on the day before she died. A perpetually anxious and worried woman who had borne the weight of mothering my father, her only child, during the constant uncertainty of the Great Depression, and who had experienced the trauma of being burned out of her home during those same years, suddenly became someone quite different than the one I'd known all my life. Miraculously relieved of the terrible, ceaseless burdens of memory and the ravages of her final illness, something was visited upon her, something undeniable. Evident to her and to others, she was lifted, maybe even resurrected. At last, she actually shimmered as the truth of her made itself known. It may have been the first time I ever saw her genuinely smile. In retrospect, it was as if she was trying on her new life.

I've witnessed this same kind of shifting in others to varying degrees, and it has always impressed me as a kind of farewell to what they thought they were, a welcoming of their encroaching new reality. It's as if the ego finally surrenders, knowing the jig is up. Though not yet ready to leave entirely, in its wisdom it realizes the need for vigilance is fading. In that stepping aside of personality, truth prevails.

During the brief time between Kenny's diagnosis and his liminal experience the night before he died, I remember how he had quickly become far more accepting of life; ironically, something with which he had struggled for so long. It did not strike me as mere fatigue or resignation, but more an embracing infused with genuine peace and equanimity, a condition that had proved elusive for him before this. I couldn't help but notice how his rough edges had smoothed, his anxiety and cynicism abated. As his end came near, he was gently facing this sum of all human fear under an influence of grace.

It was shortly after the time during my father's final hospitalization when I had told him he would soon die, that we had a conversation with a hospice nurse. I'd first noticed the change about him when I walked into his room that day. His eyes had never looked as bright and clear, or as blue. A warm, easy smile and cheerful disposition greeted me. His color was improved from the previous evening's visit, and his hair was combed. He looked refreshed. I could not recall having seen him appear this way in quite some time, maybe ever. It was as if I could see into the center of him, the dense opacity of his personality dissolved at last. Even the air around him seemed more alive. He looked like his mother had 40 years before.

I brought him by wheelchair to the conference room where we were to meet. The nurse was there to assess him holistically, and he, never one to subscribe to such notions, cooperated magnificently. In fact, he began by flirting with her. She introduced herself as Rose, was a bit older than me, a bit younger than he, and was possessed of a warm personality and beautiful smile. There was an element of the absurd in seeing this man, clearly at the end of his life engaging in such a way, but it was actually fun to watch. She played along kindly. Even as we moved toward discussing more pertinent matters such as his looming death, he continued to be lucid and of good cheer, generous, graceful, and accepting.

After some time, he began to tire, so I brought him back to his room. As he eased into bed, I told him I was going back for some more conversation with our new friend Rose. Previously, he would have been suspicious and questioning about this, but as he took off his glasses and settled in, he told me that sounded wonderful and to let him know how things turned out. I think he may have dozed off even before I left his room.

Leaning forward in her seat as I returned, Rose greeted me with a pointed question. "So. What did you think of that?"

"I think he is going to die very soon," I replied.

She seemed to relax at this, smiling a little. "I agree with you. It's good you can see that," she said.

The onset of his passing began on the following day.

As I reflect on these various experiences of death's approach, it would be easy to conclude this occurs only in certain instances where the circumstances are gentle, and the end is clearly in sight. But what of something more sudden or violent? What if the end comes by one's own hand in an act of suicide, for example? What then?

My son's name is Keith. Only as I write now does it occur to me that I had not yet mentioned it in this work. How odd it is that I should have neglected the name attached to such a cataclysmic life, a life that ended in such horror. Were he observing me, I would imagine he'd say something dry. Something like, "About time." I know he'd appreciate a discussion of something sweet about him. He'd want it known there was more to it at the end than all the horror.

During my second marriage, I was blessed with a beautiful father-in-law. But just as our marriage was beginning to show signs of its own imminent end, he died in a virtual hail of grace, an extended and quite perfect version of what I've been describing. After the funeral, our family gathered in his back yard under the shade of an old maple and had the kind of time he would have loved. Keith was with us. He'd insisted upon it, for even though he was not a blood relation, he genuinely loved the old man.

At the time he was living in some kind of a program, one designed to assist those with addiction and mental health difficulties. He'd landed there after the latest in a long series of life crises. It could be said his overall condition at the time was labile—depending on his medication status and the current state of his sobriety, one never knew how he would be. There was always a measure of apprehension connected with the prospect of being with him. Yet the idea of excluding him from this gathering, of denying him connection with his family, would have been unthinkable. We hoped for the best, and made arrangements for him to join us.

One of his stepsisters had brought him. She discreetly mentioned to me that he "seems really good today." I observed him as he moved through us all. He was warm and engaging, clear eyed and articulate, happy to be with everyone. His lightly sardonic humor was evident, yet juxtaposed with a genuine and tender kindness, and all of his interactions left behind a trail of hope for his future. It was mine to bring him back to his program afterward; he'd needed to make curfew. As he made the rounds through his family to say goodbye, he told each of them how he loved them and how much they meant to him. It was the last time most would see him. Less than three months later, it ended.

Our ride back was subdued yet comfortable, and most of what he had to say came from a place of gratitude. I don't remember all the details of our quiet conversation, but I wish I did. I know it left me feeling better about his chances and thankful for the day we had just shared. I would see him one more time before the end, but how he was on this particular day is a better memory for me. Now, as I recall him walking away from the car, I'm drawn back to that rear seat of our beautiful canoe where I'm watching him paddle, the pristine, sun-dappled river is before him, he's happy to be where he is, and we are both mercifully blind to the future. It is as if no time has passed since.

When the inexperienced view this sort of thing, they're often confused. It appears to be an impossibility, a reversal of fortune that defies reality. I have heard it referred to by some as the last hurrah, but this strikes me as an arrogant and vulgar term meant to dismiss humanity in its closest proximity to the mystical. In truth, it is reality shining through, a way to glimpse the far country, our true home, while still of the earth; a way to know there is so much more. It is a gift that extends from the dying through to the living, a gift that points toward something new and wonderful, something unchanging which is forever, and which has always been. The next time I'm around for a moment like this, I think it will be best for me to say I was able to truly know this person at last.

As I find myself in the place of pondering this shift from the human experience to that which follows, I'm led to consider some more possibilities. Perhaps it is that we might just be an ephemeral shimmering on the entire expanse of life itself, a twinkling of reflected sunlight on some distant ocean wave rolling toward shore, and that the whole brilliant world and everything in it is a shimmering too. I've wondered if it's true that from some no-place outside of time, we've been dropped through a holy instant into time and place—yet only a pale reflection, an image of what eternity looks like through the limited creations of time, where the world now can only appear as a mere shadow of what it truly is. In eternity, a flashing shimmer. In time, some measure of days; maybe tens of thousands, maybe not. Could it be that in all this time of ours, we have lived perfectly insulated, shielded from a reality that is closer than breath yet simply not possible to grasp as sensate beings?

And maybe it is that we do not so much come into this world, as out of it—that our lives are exhaled into being by God Itself.

After all, our bodies are made of stardust. And when our time has run its course, perhaps we find ourselves inhaled, back into the unseen, the forever, the all of it—taken up and made whole again. Yet maybe too, after we do pass, though no longer of form, our essence may remain as a soft memory, as a voice on a warm breeze, as a gentle current on some peaceful river.

> The water flows
> along its course
> a flat current through stream or river.
> Always water.
> Until a whirlpool takes form,
> who knows why or how?
> Maybe the water just wants to spin and dance a while.
> But from the always-water
> comes a swirling for a time,
> and then something changes
> who knows why or how?
> Maybe the water wishes some rest.
> And the whirlpool dissolves

back to the flat current

of the always-water.

Around the bends

and over the rocks

and under the keels

of beautiful canoes.

* * *

And yet. No matter how evolved our view of death may become, no matter how sudden and shocking, or benevolent and loving, even as sweet as anyone's passing may appear to be as the end of their suffering, there is the sense of immutable loss that becomes the lot of those who remain in what can feel like an unbearable void. Moments of yearning string along endlessly into the hours, the days, the months, the years, the remainder of a life. How to be with this? How to be? How to be with such abiding grief?

The person we love maybe most in the world has just died. Left us forever and forever, and forever more. Dissolved like a vapor, quintessence of the ephemeral. Like a smoke ring floating across a room, then loosening, then shapeless, then just air. We may begin to call to them and our voice catches and nothing comes out. After all, who would answer? Raise our hand to touch? The same. The hand will linger a moment, then fall with the remembering. "Oh yes," we'll say. "Not here."

In a hundred ways it is the remembering; something left on the fireplace mantle, on a hanger in the closet, a bookmark left on an end table, their favorite food seen at the grocery and almost purchased. We notice how much lonelier the old clock's ticking sounds in the middle of the night, and the faint scent remaining in a pillow or a baby's blanket. The simple rituals of the day, now performed in ways that speak of absence. We notice how quiet it's become, and how quiet it needs to be. We see our beloved everywhere and in everything, even sometimes in a stranger's face. Remembering proves to be as persistent as breathing. Often, at the oddest moments, we find ourselves shaking our head ever so slightly in disbelief, yet knowing it really is true. But regardless of the nature of the relationship now changed forever, it often seems to come down to time, for memory is a function that can only work in time. And how much time did we have? Not enough. That is precisely how much. Perhaps this is near the root of the matter. What is remembered? The past. And when is it remembered? Right now. Of course. Only now.

This is when ritual begins. Perhaps a candle is lit in some room, dark and silent as it is empty of the one so missed, and the mind commences to spin the holy tales of a time when life could move beyond the globe of a candle's glow. Remembering is a movement, after all. Have to start somewhere. All that's needed now, we think, is a moth. Cliché maybe, but what else could so rightly punctuate a moment like this? The candle burns. The memories arrive as does the distant rumbling of a late day storm in summer. We notice as it rolls along, growing closer. The regrets and joys, the sins of omission and commission, things that were said, things left unsaid, the rumbling. Deeper we notice, and deeper still. The ritual repeats, the time does pass. In a while, maybe a little less the heart aches, a little less to weep, or maybe not. Something moving, though. And then one day a thought may come to help us through—an epiphany courtesy of abiding grief. If its naked anguish can be relieved, even if but for a moment, and grief can find itself welcomed whole, maybe even called our friend, it may reveal at last a tender mercy, and we creatures of time can begin to see that a prayer is afoot. Now, from somewhere out of candlelit prayers of remembering and noticing, we may even hear a whispered intimation that grief cannot possibly live without the love that delivered it.

Wouldn't it be that love is the answer after all? What else in heaven's name could it ever be? How to love the one no longer here? How to love anything that has passed forever from view? Love known by its new name; love now known as Grief, a love colored with compassionate tenderness for ourselves and others. Imagine that.

With anything that ever began, its ending was always assured. This, the soul knows is the truth of its earthly life, even if the mind or heart chooses to forget. Nothing is exempt. This is what was agreed upon. What would better assure our innate love of life, our hunger for experience, the imperative to breathe? It's time that fools the heart into believing that forever belongs here. To know, to love anyone or anything means to love the end as well, to love it like a soul would, like a heart really can't, to love the end of what began as the very continuation of its essence.

A grieving candle's glow. A room so quiet, so empty. A doorway to pass through. A pointer to follow. Other kinds of love remembered there too. The first love—a gaze into mother's eyes, something to hold onto in the great confusion of arrival—a lifeline. All the different ways of love that followed this one, all showing the same thing: something collapsing, the space between everyone and everything crumbling, all things becoming one thing. Like a soul would. Like a heart can't. That it had to be the pain to see it as true. That it had to be the pain to show the way.

Life is echoing against itself now beyond the quiet, empty room. Life and death, grief as love; all are at it still, colliding in a swirling vortex of a dance set to a lilting, echoing rhapsody beneath a sparsely clouded night sky, and all under the watch of a plump, gibbous moon. They're holding tight, invoking the pain, gaining some serious attention, refusing to let go of each other. There's been an agreement about this for the longest time, since things began, since things have ended. The prayer has been afoot.

* * *

The great teachers will one day stand down from time, for it is time's nature to expire. But on some distant morning, when dim, early light peeks over the horizon and gently summons the body from its dreaming, from all the loves known there, the terrors too, some moments of that world that will linger awhile, remembered; moments to dissolve in the stretch and yawn and the first noise lifting from the throat: a mourning noise, a declaration. And as the waking life encroaches, memory may falter as to the particulars, but essence...essence will live forever, even beyond any worldly notion of what forever means.

AFTERWORD

How often have we been delivered to a moment, a relationship, or a circumstance where there can simply be no doubt that it was the threads of our past that led us to it, and which made our presence essential to what followed? Life has a way of weaving, layering, and coloring its fabric, keeping us essentially clueless until it comes time for us to step back and take in the divine tapestry—see it more fully and in its perfection, and see too the hand of grace that is undeniable, a grace which was there from the beginning. Of course, those moments, relationships, and circumstances are not stand-alone pieces, but are themselves woven into something infinite and so often incomprehensible. To really understand would require transcendence, and in my own modest experience this has occurred mostly in lovely, unforgettable, and transient flashes. Such is life—an ongoing cycle of transcendence and return.

We are drawn to another for so many reasons. I don't believe it is ever just one or even a simple handful. But there are those relationships that force the attention and encourage our focus.

There are some that may serve to remind us there is more going on than the obvious, and that our path through life is not capricious. Tracing their true beginnings will always lead back to a place just beyond memory's reach, just beyond time itself. I suppose one must begin somewhere, though.

* * *

She and I and I first met as friends, part of a circle of people who gathered for the purpose of finding a spiritual solution to the matters of life. We quickly determined that we had something in common—both of our sons who were of similar age had each been living a life of severe chemical addiction. We had progressed in our respective relationships with Keith and J. to where we no longer recognized our boys. Everything observable about them had been so radically distorted, they had become complete strangers to us. In a very real sense, we had the full experience of their loss, yet without their physical deaths to show for it.

A few years after we first met, my son's life journey ended. She had found out about it from mutual friends, and I saw her next at his wake. After greeting me, she went to the casket and I took notice as she regarded Keith's body. I knew with absolute certainty that the body she saw was J.'s. Her face reflected grief's timeless nature.

In the aftermath of his death, we became closer and eventually fell into a committed relationship. Beyond our clear and obvious attraction, our shared grief was always present, an essential connecting point, a wordless place. Among the unspoken thoughts between us was the unsustainable nature of her son's life as he was continuing to live it.

Though my dear one never had the opportunity to know Keith, coincidence did allow me to have known J. even before she and I had come to know each other more closely. Her son and I shared several conversations over time. The elusive nature of his sobriety often came up, and I always found it disturbing how casually he would acknowledge the overwhelming nature of his problems, how resigned he'd become, and how resistant to a solution he seemed to be. I would often recall the same kinds of conversations I'd had with Keith, and though I tended to keep it to myself, there was a looming sense of hopelessness.

Years passed. During that time, my partner would often wonder when her turn would come to experience the remainder of her grief. The phone might ring a certain way, perhaps a missed call would come without a message, or a piece would appear in the news about the epidemic of opioid poisoning deaths—deaths which usually happened to those who were alone. On some days her anxiety about this would peak; her first waking thought would ask the question: Is this the day? It was a question that burned into her, a reflex, a recurring, waking nightmare. Though hope remained for his recovery, J. rarely showed an interest in any other answer than the one he'd found, rarely showed signs of the self-compassion required to want something better. His chances dwindled as more time passed. As my son had taught me so well, it was about a pain that nothing else could touch.

Pain untransformed will always become pain passed on. It is as inevitable as electricity finding the way to ground. The day finally came. I went to her immediately, my purpose as clear as the path which had spirited me along from a weighted delivery room in 1981. I recognized her now as one of my own—it's always this thing in the eyes.

That day, in shock after hearing of her son's death, she kept repeating the answer to her oft asked, burned in question. Hearing this, I could offer little else but a kind hand and some hard-earned words to a lost boy's mom, spoken in a voice most perfectly her own:

My dearest one said…

This is the day

the day I knew would come.

The day I would join you

in the fellowship of the wrecked and devastated.

The day I'd know

the fear

the rage

the regret

the wondering that will not end.

Some days will begin with blackened thick and clotted skies

until suddenly a gentle breeze blows.

And in the holy instant it lifts,

the dawn will become a wispy pink and lovely affair

fresh and new

as I join you and say,

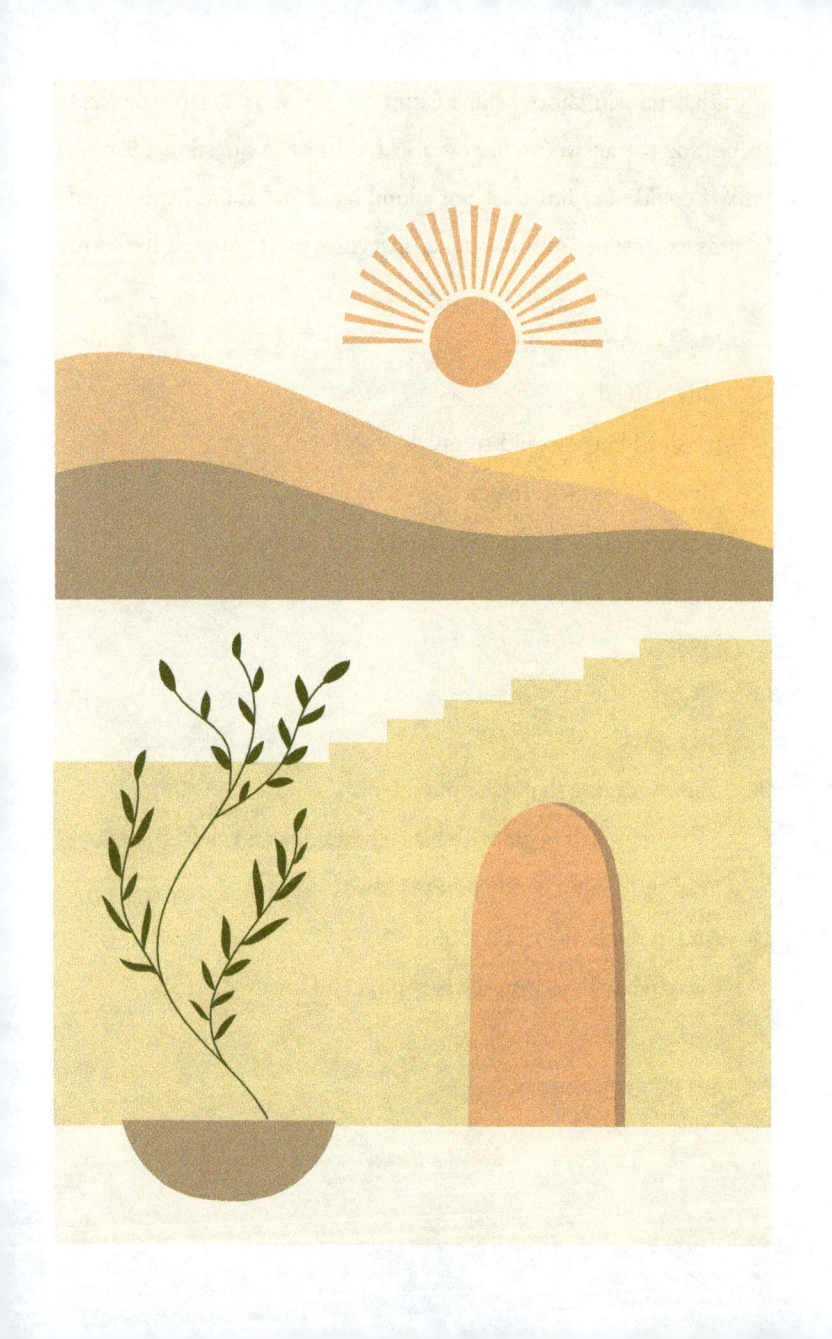

this is the day,

the day I knew would come.

The day I would join you

in the fellowship of the healed and blessed.

When I'd know

the love

the peace

the forgiveness

the wonder that will not end.

You said it would come along in waves like this

so sloppy and tangled and twisted.

You said it all belongs

and promised me all will be well

along the Way we now go.

Promised.

We will recognize the others,

see it in their eyes

always in their eyes,

the only place left to look.

Our fellows of the

wrecked and devastated and healed and blessed,

along the Way we all now go.

I may be having a dream that life will always hold a holy place where death delights to help those who remain. How often I wonder about our boys, though. Maybe there was more to this. I've noticed something in their respective childhood and more recent photos—that certain something in their eyes, something familiar, and something left unsaid, maybe a vague longing for innocence not quite forgotten, a searching. Maybe too, a tenderness of being that was much too fine and sensitive for such a coarse and terrifying world.

Neither my partner nor I had ever thought of them as having been together, because to us they seemed to be of different times, unconnected other than by the similarities in their respective circumstances. But in these photos, there was revealed a sense of brotherhood, an idea that somehow, in some place, they were a well-matched pair. To me, there was a seamlessness in the experience she and I had shared, which was now more apparent as I considered these images of J. and Keith. It all flowed together. Us. Our boys. One thing. The almost nine years between their deaths, now compressed into no time at all.

Shortly after Keith had died, I was sifting through his social media for the first time and saw a name and face I recognized. Turns out their paths had crossed years before in a treatment facility and they'd become casual friends, never having been aware of their parents' acquaintance. Even though at the time the full implication of this could not yet have been apparent, I knew then I'd been delivered by a moment when the hand of grace was plainly in sight, in a moment out of time, where death had indeed delighted to help the living.

Although we are no longer joined as a couple, and despite our difficulties, I believe we had been delivered to a shared sacrament, a high and holy purpose, its unfolding seen most clearly in retrospect, for to share the grief of lost children with another can be little else than a calling.

With all of it, I remain wondering. I will always wonder.

ACKNOWLEDGMENTS

Tom Lagasse, the Max Perkins of my writing life. Beyond wonderful.

First readers and sanity checkers: Bill Considine, Nancy DePecol, Terri DeMontrond, Terri Dyer, Bill Ludwig, Rick Ludwig, Lynn Martin, Dianne Slater.

The inspiring dreams of Gerard.

David K. Leff. For having been here.

Leslie M. Browning, my publisher. Again.

The whirlpool metaphor used in the poem *Always Water* is attributed to Bernardo Kastrup.

The All of it, in all of it. For everything.

ABOUT THE AUTHOR

Stephen Drew lives in a bucolic lakeside community in northwestern Connecticut. In addition to *Around the Forever Bend,* he also authored the memoir *Into the Thin: A Pilgrimage Walk Across Northern Spain* which was his first published work. Stephen practices a minimalist lifestyle which includes daily walking, mostly on the roads and paths near his home. Hiking there and elsewhere serves as a centerpiece of contemplative living and an ongoing connection to Source. He currently resides in Morris, Connecticut. Visit him at authorstephendrew.com.

WAYFARER

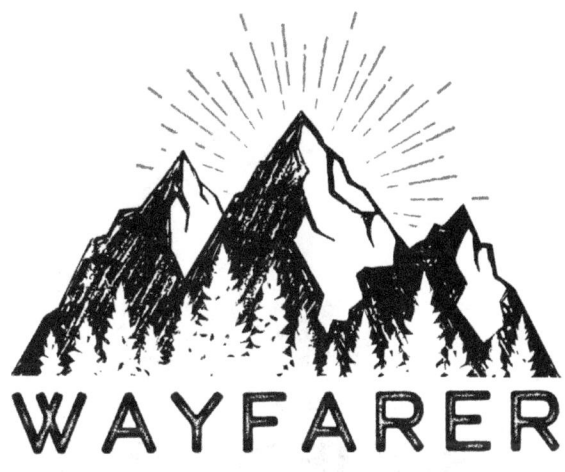

BASED IN THE BERKSHIRE MOUNTAINS, MASS.

The Wayfarer Magazine. Since 2012, *The Wayfarer* has been offering literature, interviews, and art with the intention to inspires our readers, enrich their lives, and highlight the power for agency and change-making that each individual holds. By our definition, a wayfarer is one whose inner-compass is ever-oriented to truth, wisdom, healing, and beauty in their own wandering. The Wayfarer's mission as a publication is to foster a community of contemplative voices and provide readers with resources and perspectives that support them in their own journey.

Wayfarer Books is our newest imprint! After nearly 10 years in print, *The Wayfarer Magazine* is branching out from our magazine to become a full-fledged publishing house offering full-length works of eco-literature!

Wayfarer Farm & Retreat is our latest endeavor, springing up in the Berkshire Mountains of Massachusetts. Set to open to the public in 2024, the 15 acre retreat will offer workshops, farm-to-table dinners, off-grid retreat cabins, and artist residencies.

WWW.WAYFARERBOOKS.ORG

HOMEBOUND
PUBLICATIONS

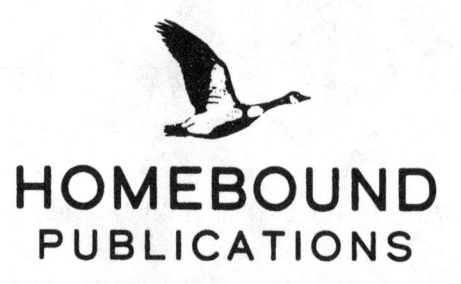

Since 2011 We are an award-winning independent publisher striving to ensure that the mainstream is not the only stream. More than a company, we are a community of writers and readers exploring the larger questions we face as a global village. It is our intention to preserve contemplative storytelling. We publish full-length introspective works of creative non-fiction, literary fiction, and poetry.

Look for Our Imprints Little Bound Books, Owl House Books, The Wayfarer Magazine, Wayfarer Books & Navigator Graphics

HOMEBOUNDPUBLICATIONS.COM

LITTLE BOUND BOOKS

Little Bound Books is an imprint of Homebound Publications
devoted to short form fiction and creative nonfiction.
Our books are small enough to slip in your back pocket
but powerful enough to leave an impact.

LITTLEBOUNDBOOKS.COM